I0439784

DIY Bath Salt Recipes

The Ideal Therapeutic Hobby or Gift

Contents

Copyright

contained within is the solitary and utter responsibility of the recipient reader. Under no circumstances will any legal responsibility or blame be held against the publisher for any reparation, damages, or monetary loss due to the information herein, either directly or indirectly.
Respective authors own all copyrights not held by the publisher.

The information herein is offered for informational purposes solely, and is universal as so. The presentation of the information is without contract or any type of guarantee assurance.

The trademarks that are used are without any consent, and the publication of the trademark is without permission or backing by the trademark owner. All trademarks and brands within this book are for clarifying purposes only and are the owned by the owners themselves, not affiliated with this document.

Introduction

I want to thank you and congratulate you for downloading the book, *"DIY Bath Salts Recipes"*. This book contains proven steps and strategies on how to make bath salts.

Bath salts are often used for therapeutic and medicinal purposes. Bath salts are water soluble materials that are either added to the bath water or rubbed directly on the skin.

Commercial bath salts tend to be overpriced considering how easy it is to make your own. There are a lot of ingredients that you can use to make your own bath salt. You can create your own essential oil blend and even add herbs and spices. The best thing about making your own bath salts is that you can customize it depending on your needs.

Since bath salts have many benefits, you may even be tempted to make a lot of varieties. This book contains a lot of bath salt recipes that can suit your mood. It also has recipes on bath salts that provide therapeutic benefits.

Lastly, you can make bath salts and give them away as gifts. It is economical compared to other gifts, but it will not look cheap especially if you pack it properly in a cute bottle. People generally enjoy receiving handmade gifts and appreciate the effort that was put into it.

Thanks again for downloading this book, I hope you enjoy it!

Chapter 1 - Bath Salts

Bath salts are water soluble materials that have the same appearance and texture as salt. Bath salts are popularly used in spa and wellness centers. They come in different scents and some have therapeutic and healing properties as well.

Benefits of Bath Salts

Relaxation benefit

One of the main reasons why people use bath salts is that it helps relieve stress after a long day. Bath salts contain magnesium that can drain stress from the body. It can also increase your adrenaline level and boost your mood.

The magnesium in the salt is absorbed in the skin and helps produce serotonin that creates a feeling of relaxation and calmness. Studies show that it can also increase stamina by stimulating the ATP that refers to energy packets in the cells. Health and wellness experts say that using bath salt three times in a week can help you look and feel better.

Relives pain

A salt bath can reduce muscle pain and inflammation. It is a great treatment for headache, asthma and sore muscles. Some people soak their feet into warm water and add bath salts to relieve any pain. The salt can also soften the skin and make it easier to exfoliate.

Helps nerves function properly

Studies show that bath salts can regulate electrolytes in the body. This ensures proper circulation in the nerves. Some bath salts, especially those that contain magnesium, play an important role in the absorption of calcium which is the main conductor of nerves in the body.

Beauty benefits

Soaking in water with bath salts can instantly give you smooth skin. The texture of the salt can gently exfoliate the top layer of the skin. It can also improve circulation which helps prevent cellulites and stretch marks.

Eliminates toxins from the body

The minerals in the salt are easily absorbed in the body. It can remove dirt, oil and pollution in the pores through a process known as reverse osmosis which is pulling the salt from the body and taking the toxins with it.

What to consider

You should consider your skin type when selecting ingredients for your bath salts. You can also select bath salts depending on your needs. Lavender bath salts are suitable if you want to relieve while tangerine bath salts can improve your mood and increase energy.

How to use bath salts

Bath salts are not only easy to make, they are also very easy to use. Although the most popular way to use these salts is for bathing, you can also use them as a scrub or cleanser.

Bath salts come in different colors and textures. Colored bath salts will change the color of your bath water, but will not taint you skin. You can choose bath salt that matches your mood or what you'll like your mood to be. Blue can be very soothing while bright colors can invigorate you when you are feeling sluggish. The texture of the salt can also vary. Large grain salts take a bit longer to dissolve while smaller bath salts are gentle enough for exfoliation.

To use, simply add a few tablespoons of bath salts and stir the water with your hand. The fragrance of the salt will be released with the steam. You can also directly rub the bath salt into your skin or add a little amount of water to make it easier to apply into skin.

Chapter 2 - Types of Salt to Use

Bath salts typically require a few ingredients. There are many options when it comes to the types of salts that you can use. You can also include 'salt' ingredients that are chemically different from the ones that you add to your food. Iodized salt is a refined salt variety and has a trace amount of iodine. It is finely grounded. Although iodized salt is the most common salt found in households, it is rarely used in bath salts since it may trigger allergic reaction for people with sensitive skin.

Here are some of the salts used in making bath salts:

Ancient Sea Salt
Sea salt deposits formed in mountain ranges for over 150 million years. These salts are carefully harvested. The salt contains about 84 trace minerals that give it a beautiful pink color.

Atlantic Sea Salt
The Atlantic sea salt is collected from deep waters by drying sea water into large trays and letting it evaporate naturally. This type of sea salt is great for adding color or scent since it is absorbent. Atlantic sea salt comes in different sizes.

Coarse Salt
Coarse salt is usually 2-3 millimeters in size. It can also absorb coloring and scents easily. Coarse

salt is ideal for making salt potpourri.

Crystal Salt
Crystal salts are large chunks of salt that are great to add in potpourri bags. You hang it in the spout of the faucet and let the water run over the salt. You can also add herbs and oil to increase its therapeutic benefits.

Dead Sea Salt
Dead sea salt is very famous for its beauty benefit. It is different from other salts because of its mineral content. It only has 8% sodium chloride content, but has a high magnesium, potassium and sulfate content. Dead sea salt can help with skin conditions like eczema and psoriasis. It can also reduce pain and inflammation. Its mineral content is credited for its detoxification benefit.

Dendritic Salt
Dendritic salt is purified sodium chloride that is crystallized. It is very absorbent and can hold on to fragrances, making it a great choice if you want to add essential oils. It is also used as a preservative in many sea salt blends.

Epsom Salt
Epsom salt is actually pure magnesium that is in a crystal form. However, unlike regular salt, it does not have sodium sulfate. Epsom salt has many therapeutic and medicinal benefits and can relieve health problems like joint pain, digestive problem and chronic fatigue.

European Spa Salt
European salt is harvested similar to Atlantic salt. It can be added to your bath water directly. It is usually available in two varieties: fine and coarse. Fine grain salt is perfect for exfoliation while coarse salt is ideal for therapeutic blends.

Gray Bath Salt
Gray bath salt is usually harvested in France. Its gray color is indicative of its trace minerals absorbed from the sea. This type of sea salt is unwashed and unrefined so it retains all of the nutrients that are vital to the human body.

Hawaiian Red Salt
Hawaiian red bath salt is also known as Alaea salt. This natural salt gets its reddish hue from red clay. Volcanic red clay is high in iron oxide and is beneficial in healing wounds and muscle pains.

Solar Sea Salt
Solar salt is a term used to define salt that has been dried under the sun. It has large crystals that look very beautiful when mixed with finer salt like Epsom salt.

Sulfur Salt
Sulfur salt or Indian black salt has a pink-gray color that is very popular in Japan, France and Spain. It was used to treat inflammation and respiratory problems because of its antiseptic properties. The sulfur salt is naturally harvested in India and Pakistan.

Chapter 3 - Calming & Moisturizing Salts

Soaking in a tub filled with warm water and bath salt can help drain your stress away.   Make these soothing bath salts whenever you feel the need to calm down and unwind.

Sweet Lavender Bath Salt

Ingredients:
2 cups Epsom salt
25 ml sunflower oil
Few lavender flowers or leaves
25 ml lavender oil
Natural purple food coloring
Makes enough for 2 baths

Procedure:
Rub the lavender leaves to release their oil and fragrance. Combine the salt and leaves in a bowl. Add the oils and water. Stir in the coloring. Make sure to distribute the color evenly. Scoop the mixture into your jar. Use one cup for every bath. Make sure that it is dissolved properly before you soak your body.

Rose Milk Bath Salt

Ingredients:
½ cup Epsom salt
Red food coloring
1 ½ cups powdered milk (full fat)
½ cup dried rose petals
7 drops essential oil
Makes enough for 2 baths

Procedure:
Combine the powdered milk and Epsom salt in a bowl. Add the coloring and stir until it has a nice pink color. Add the rose essential oil. Pour it into your desired packaging.

Valentine Bath Salt

Ingredients:
3 cups Epsom salt
1 cup baking soda
2 cups sea salt of choice
5 drops lavender oil
5 drops chamomile oil
Red food coloring
Makes enough for 3 baths

Procedure:
Combine the sea salt and Epsom in a bowl. Make sure that the mixture is as smooth as possible so break down any clumps using a spoon or your fingers. Add the oils then stir the mixture. Continue to add the oil until you achieve your desired fragrance. Add the coloring until you have a pinkish shade. Stir the mixture then pour in a jar.

Brown Vanilla Bath Salt

Ingredients:
30 ml grape seed oil
½ cup Epsom Salt
¾ cup sea salt of choice
1 tbsp vanilla essence
Makes enough for 1 bath

Procedure:
Combine the salts in a bowl. Add a few drops of the oils gradually. Stir and make sure that the oil is evenly distributed. Store it in a glass jar.

Frankincense Bath Salt

Ingredients:
2 cups Epsom salt
20 drops Frankincense essential oil
Makes enough for 2 baths

Procedure:
Combine the salt and oil. Make sure to break up any lumps that may form. Pour in a jar.

Calming Bath Salt

Ingredients:
1 cup sea salt
6 drops geranium oil
2 drops rosewood oil
6 drops rose essential oil
6 drops lavender oil
Makes enough for 1 bath

Procedure:
Add the oil to the salt one drop at a time. Stir the mixture so that the oil distributes evenly.

Exotic Calming Bath Salts

Ingredients:
1 cup Dead Sea salt
3 drops roman chamomile
1 drop jasmine oil
1 drop rose
3 drops ylang ylang oil

Procedure:
Combine the ingredients in a cup or bowl. Make sure to stir gently. Pour in your bath water and soak for 15-25 minutes.

Soothing Oatmeal Bath Salt

Ingredients:
1 cup sea salt
1/2 oz lavender oil
2 cups Epsom salt
1 ½ cup oatmeal, pulverized
Makes enough for 3 baths

Procedure:
Measure the ingredients carefully and make sure to break up any clumps that may form. Make sure that you grind the oatmeal until it is very fine and has the same texture as sugar. Add the essential oil. Stir the ingredients together and pack into jars.

Peaceful Bath Salt
Ingredients:
½ cup sea salt of choice
6 drops ylang ylang oil
6 drops jasmine oil
6 drops rose oil
Makes enough for 1 bath

Procedure:
Add the essential oils one drop at a time. Stir the mixture together and break any lumps that may form.

Warming Bath Salt

Ingredients:
6 drops tangerine oil
4 drops cinnamon lea oil
2 drops lavender oil
1 cup sea salt of choice
  Drops ginger oil
6 drops clove bud oil
Makes enough for 1 bath

Procedure:
Combine the ingredients in a bowl. Stir everything until you reach the desired scent. Pour in your bath water then stir.

Lavender and Green Tea Bath Salt

Ingredients:
1 cup Epsom salt
15 drops lavender oil
2 tbsp green tea leaves, loose
Makes enough for 1 bath

Procedure:
Add the lavender oil to the sea salt. Stir to combine. Crush the green tea leaves until it is very fine. Add to the salt mixture. Stir before you add it to your bath water.

Lavender and Tea Tree Bath Salt

Ingredients:
10 drops lavender oil
1 cup sea salt
10 drops tea tree oil
Makes enough for 1 bath

Procedure:
Add the oil to the salt. Stir until combined. Make sure that there are no clumps of salt. Add to your desired container or pour it in your bath water.

Renew and Relax Bath Salts

Ingredients:
½ cup sea salt of choice
½ cup Epsom salt
4 drops sandalwood oil
8 drops jasmine oil
4 drops ylang ylang oil
Makes enough for 1 bath

Procedure:
Combine the salts in a bowl. Add the essential oils and stir with a spoon. Pour into your bath water and stir the mixture until it dissolves. Soak for 20 minutes until you are relaxed.

Rosemary and Cranberry Bath Salt

Ingredients:
6 drops rosemary oil
1 cup sea salt
18 drops cranberry oil
Makes enough for 1 bath
Procedure:
Add the essential oils to the salt. Store the mixture in a small pack or use immediately.

Chamomile Bath Salts

Ingredients:
1 cup Epsom salt
10 drops chamomile oil
5 drops lavender oil
Makes enough for 1 bath

Procedure:
Combine the ingredients in a bowl. Stir then pour in water or store in a package.

Chapter 4 - Energizing & Invigorating Salts

Earthy Bath Salt

Ingredients:
6 drops germanium oil
6 drops rosewood oil
1 cup Epsom salt
4 drops rosemary oil
Makes enough for 1 bath

Procedure:
Combine the ingredients in a bowl Stir the mixture until the fragrance is well distributed. Pour into your bath water.

Energizing Citrus Bath Salt

Ingredients:
½ cup sea salt of choice
1 cup Epsom salt
6 drops tangerine oil
4 drops grapefruit oil
4 drops lemon oil
8 drops sweet orange oil
Makes enough for 2 baths

Procedure:
Add the essential oils in the salt combination. Stir the mixture until the oil is well distributed. Pour in a container or into you bath water.

Stimulating Bath Salt

Ingredients:
1 cup sea salt of choice
4 drops rosemary oil
6 drops lemon oil
4 drops geranium oil
8 drops lavender oil
Makes enough for 1 bath

Procedure:
Pour the salt in a bowl then add the essential oil one drop at a time. Stir the mixture until the fragrance is incorporated. Let it dissolve in your bath water. Soak for 10-20 minutes. This is best used in the morning.

Uplifting Bath Salt

Ingredients:
1 cup Atlantic sea salt
46 drops ylang ylang oil
6 drops sandalwood oil
6 drops patchouli oil
Makes enough for 1 bath

Procedure:
Combine the oil in a bowl and pour over the salt. Stir the mixture quickly and break any lumps that may form. Pour in your bath water.

Rosemary Salt Bath

Ingredients:
2 cups Epsom salt
2 drops red food coloring
2 tbsp baking soda
4 drops rosemary oil
Makes enough for 2 baths

Procedure:
Combine the baking soda and Epsom salt in a bowl. Add the oil then stir the ingredients. Add the rosemary oil. Stir in the mixture into your bath water. Soak for a few minutes.

Rainbow Bath Salt

Ingredients:
2 cups Dead Sea salt
3 different food coloring
5 ml citrus essential oil
Makes enough for 2 baths

Procedure:
Scoop the salt into three Ziploc bags. Add food coloring into each bag. Add 1-3 drops of essential oils in each bag. Shake the bags until the ingredients are mixed inside. Add another drop of the essential oil and stir. Pour the first color in a jar. Layer the next colors until you have a rainbow effect. This bath salt is a great gift or party favor.

Mint Mojito Bath Salt

Ingredients:
2 cups Epsom salt
10 drops mint essential oil
3 drops green food coloring
1 cup mint, finely diced
Juice and zest of 1 lime
Makes enough for 4 baths

Procedure:
Combine the mint, lime juice, lime zest and salt in a bowl. Stir the mixture using a spoon. Add the mint essential oil.   Stir in the food coloring. Stir the mixture until the color and fragrance is well distributed. You can use ½ cup for each bath.

Lemon Almond Salt Bath

Ingredients:
10 drops almond oil
2 cup sea salt of choice
10 drops lemon oil
Makes enough for 2 baths

Procedure:
Combine all of the ingredients in a bowl. Break off any lumps then transfer it in a container or pour it in a tub.

Orange Dream Bath Salts

Ingredients:
3 cups Epsom salt
3 tbsp glycerin
1 tsp orange extract
1 tsp vanilla extract
12 drops red food coloring
50 drops yellow food coloring
Makes enough for 2 baths

Procedure:
Place 2 cups of glycerin in a bowl. Add in 2 cups of salt and stir well until the ingredients are combined. Mix the red food coloring and stir the ingredients until it has a nice orange color. Make the vanilla salts. Combine one cup of Epsom salt with 1 tbsp of glycerin. Add the vanilla extract and stir the mixture. Make sure to break off any lumps that may form. Layer the orange and white colored salt in a glass jar. This creates a wonderful layering effect.

Grapefruit Bath Salt

Ingredients:
1 cup Atlantic sea salt
4 drops grapefruit oil
2 drops purple food coloring
Makes enough for 1 bath

Procedure:
Pour the salt in a bowl. Add the food coloring into the salt. Mix in 4 drops of the grapefruit essential oil. Transfer the mixture in a bag then shake until everything is well incorporated. Pour it in a jar or dump it directly to your bath tub. Dissolve in water before soaking in.

Lemon Rosemary Bath Salts

Ingredients:
2 cups Epsom salt
3 tbsp fresh rosemary, chopped
2 drops blue food coloring
8 drops rosemary essential oil
½ cup baking soda
Makes enough for 2 baths

Procedure:
Mix the baking soda and Epsom salt. Add half of the oil. Stir for a few seconds then add the remaining essential oil. Chop the rosemary and zest. Add to the mixture then stir until combined. Transfer the mixture in a container.

Eucalyptus and Vanilla Bath Salts

Ingredients:
1 cup Epsom Salt
3 drops eucalyptus oil
½ cup baking soda
8 drops jojoba oil
Green food coloring
Makes enough for 2 baths

Procedure:
Pour the Epsom salt and baking soda in a large bag. Add one drop of food coloring and essential oil in the bag. Seal then shake the contents until the color is distributed evenly. Transfer in a container or use directly in your bath.

Coconut Lime Body Salt

Ingredients:
1 cup sea salt of choice
1 tbsp shredded coconut
½ cup Epsom salt
8 drops lime oil
Makes enough for 2 baths

Procedure:
Combine the Epsom and sea salt. Add the lime oil then stir the ingredients to combine. Add the shredded coconut.

Peppermint Candy Cane Salt Bath

Ingredients:
2 cups sea salt of choice
¼ cup almond oil
8 drops peppermint oil
5 drops red food coloring
Makes enough for 2 baths

Procedure:
Combine the oil to the salt. Stir the ingredients. Divide the ingredients into two bowls. Add food coloring to one bowl. Layer the red and white salts in your container. The bath salts look very pretty and are great to give as gifts

Cinnamon and Ginger Salt scrub

Ingredients:
1 cup sea salt
3 drops almond oil
1 tsp ground cinnamon
3 drops vanilla
1 tsp ground ginger
Makes enough for 2 bath salts

Procedure:
Combine all of the dry ingredients in a bowl. Add the wet ingredients and stir to combine. Transfer to your container or pour it in your bath water.

.

Chapter 5 - Medicinal & Therapeutic Salts

Back Pain Bath Salts

Ingredients:
2 cups Epsom salt
10 drops peppermint oil
5 drops rosemary oil
5 drops cinnamon oil
1 tbsp rosemary sprigs
5 drops lavender oil
1 cup bi-carb soda
5 drops eucalyptus oil
2 tbsp lavender flowers
Makes enough for 3 baths

Procedure:
Combine the salt and bi-carb soda in a large bowl. Add the essential oil and stir the mixture until the scent is distributed evenly. Add the flowers and sprigs. Transfer the mixture to the jar. Use one cup per bath and soak for 15 minutes to get the full benefits.

Aphrodisiac Bath Salt

Ingredients:
2 cups Epsom salt
½ cup baking soda
3 drops frankincense oil
1 drop cedarwood oil
1 cup Dead Sea salt
10 drops sandalwood oil
2 drops patchouli oil
6 drops red food coloring
4 drops yellow food coloring
Makes enough for 4 baths

Procedure:
Combine the baking soda and salt in a large bowl. Stir the ingredients using a spoon. Add the food coloring and essential oil. Stir the mixture using a spoon. Let the mixture cure for a day before you use it.

Muscle Mend Bath Salt

Ingredients:
3 cups Epsom salt
6 drops bergamot oil
2 drops eucalyptus oil
10 drops green food coloring
½ cup baking soda
6 drops lemongrass oil
2 drops rosemary oil
Makes enough for 3 baths

Procedure:
Pour the baking soda and salt in a bowl. Add the essential oil. Stir the mixture until the salt absorbs the oil. Mix in the coloring. Stir until the color is well distributed to the mixture. Store this in a dark jar. Let it cure for a day before using.

Stress Relief Rose Bath Salt

Ingredients:
½ cup baking soda
4 drops rose oil
1 drop vetiver oil
10 red food coloring
3 cups Dead Sea salt
6 drops palmarosa oil
4 drops rose genarium oil
1 drop ylang ylang oil
Makes enough for 4 baths

Procedure:
Mix the salt and baking soda in a bowl. Stir using a spoon. Add the oils and food coloring. Stir the mixture until the color is well distributed. Pack in a jar. Leave it for 24 hours before using.

Tension Tamer Bath Salt

Ingredients:
1 cup sea salt of choice
6 drops bergamot oil
3 drop lavender oil
2 cups Epsom salt
½ cup baking soda
6 drops sweet orange oil
Makes enough for 2 baths

Procedure:
Combine the baking soda and salt in a bowl. Stir in the essential oil until it is absorbed. Store the mixture in a dark glass. Cure for 24 hours before using.

Ginger Detox Bath

Ingredients:
2 cups Epsom salt
¼ cup ginger powder
Makes enough for 2 baths

Procedure:
Ginger powder opens up the pores and helps the body get rid of toxins. Mix the ingredients in a bowl and stir until everything is incorporated. Add one cup into your bath water and soak for at least 20 minutes to get the full benefits.

Headache Remedy Bath Salt

Ingredients:
3 cups Epsom salt
8 drops lavender oil
1 drop jasmine oil
4 drops lemon balm oil
1 drop basil oil
1 drop chamomile oil
Makes enough for 3 baths

Procedure:
Combine the oil in a bowl then slowly add it to the salt. Stir the mixture until well combined. Store the mixture in a dark glass and let it cure for a day before you use it. It is better to make this bath salt blend in advance since you need to let it cure first. Use one cup per bath.

Soothing Head Cold Bath Salt

Ingredients:
1 cup Dead Sea salt
1/4 cup dendritic salt
1 cup Epsom Salt
4 drops peppermint oil
4 drops eucalyptus oil
Makes enough for 2 baths

Procedure:
Eucalyptus can help relieve sinus congestion. Peppermint can help relieve headaches. Combine the salts in a bowl. Stir in the oil. Stir until the oils are absorbed. Pour one cup of the mixture into your bath water.

Menstrual Cramp Relief Bath Salt

Ingredients:
2 cups Epsom salt
4 drops lavender oil
2 drops chamomile oil
1 drop ginger oil
2 drops marjoram oil
3 drops geranium oil
Makes enough for 2 baths

Procedure:
Add the oils to the salt mixture. Stir until the salt absorbs the oil. Make sure that there are no lumps in the mixture. Stir it in your warm bath water. Soak for 20 minutes.

Anti-Cellulite Bath Salt Blend

Ingredients:
1 cup Dead sea salt
2 drops lemon oil
2 drops sage oil
2 drops niaouli oil
2 drops eucalyptus oil
2 drops cedarwood oil
2 drops cypress oil

Procedure:
Combine the ingredients and stir until the oil is absorbed. You can dissolve the salt in your bath water or rub it directly on your skin.

Chapter 6 - Packing your Bath Salts

Making your own bath salts is fun and convenient. It can also give you a sense of accomplishment especially after you experience the benefits of the bath salt yourself. Bath salts are great homemade gifts. You can customize the blend to suit the person you are giving the gift to. However, no matter how great your bath salt is, you still need to consider the packaging especially if you intend to give it away.

Cute containers can make your product more appealing. It also shows that you really took time and effort in making the gift. Here are some of the tips in packing your bath salts:

Use clear glass

Make your bath salt appealing by displaying it in a glass jar. Fortunately, there are many glass jars to choose from. You can choose a simple cylindrical or round jar for a classic look or choose geometrically shaped glass for something unique.

Color and layer

You can add food coloring to your bath salts to make them beautiful. If you have enough food coloring, then you can also layer different colors in a transparent container. This instantly adds a creative touch to your gift.

Place it in a bath salt bag

You can place your bath salts in individual patchouli bags. You can hang the bag in your faucet or let it soak in your bath water. Placing your bath salts in a bag is ideal if you are using large grain salts. It is also a good idea if you are adding herbs into your recipe so that you don't have to clean the tub afterwards.

Label it

You can personalize your gift by adding your own label. You can add instructions on how they can use the bath salt or even add a personal message. Be creative in designing your label. Print it in a sticker paper and cut.

Canister

Using a metal or plastic container is ideal if you are prone to breaking glass in the shower. However, you may not be able to display different colors just like in a glass container. Choose a small or medium sized canister and add a scoop in the can so that you do not wet all of the salt when using it.

Ties and twines

Tie a pretty ribbon around your container. A ribbon makes it appear more like a gift. You can have fun in using different types of ribbons and ties.

Conclusion

Thank you again for downloading this book!
I hope this book was able to help you to make therapeutic bath salts.

The next step is to try the recipes yourself.

Finally, if you enjoyed this book, then I'd like to ask you for a favor, would you be kind enough to leave a review for this book on Amazon? It'd be greatly appreciated!

Thank you and good luck!

Bonus Content

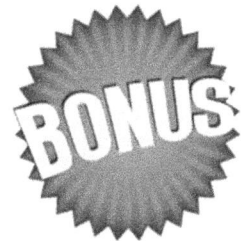

As a token of our appreciation Grand Reveur Publications would like to give you access to our exclusive bonus content (including free eBooks!).

Exclusive pre-release access to our latest eBooks Free Grand Reveur eBooks during promotional periods.

A method ANYONE can use to publish their own book and make passive income.

To receive this additional bonus content please go to the following web site:

https://ignorelimits.leadpages.net/grandreveur publications/

As this is a limited time offer it would be a shame to miss out, I recommend grabbing these bonuses before reading on